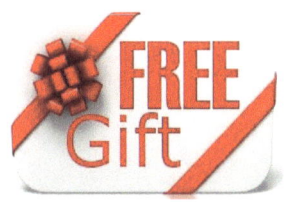

Want Priority Access to FREE eBooks Additional Materials for this Book?

As we release NEW eBooks, we offer them for FREE for a limited time. You will be the FIRST one to know when they are FREE. Join 1000's of insiders who are getting access to FREE Kindle book promotions weekly.

Click HERE for FREE additional material and FREE eBooks-
www.rictamilypublishing.com

Table of Contents

Introduction

Even though it happens to be that this is not the first time the Ebola Virus has found its way through the shores of Africa, its latest development has been that of an alarming one. As it stands now a handful of West African countries has been affected namely Guinea, Liberia, Nigeria, Senegal and Sierra Leone.

It is believed that Ebola first emerged in Sudan and Zaire in 1976. The name Ebola was named after the Zaire River called "Ebola River" The first outbreak of Ebola is said to have infected 284 people with a mortality rate of 53%. The second emergence of Ebola was reported in Yambuku, Zaire. Ebola-Zaire (EBOZ) recorded the highest mortality rate of any of the Ebola viruses (88%) infected 318 people. The third strain of Ebola, Ebola Reston (EBOR), was first identified in 1989 when infected monkeys were imported into Reston, Virginia, from Mindanao in the Philippines. Ebola has found its way in the annals of West Africa and the Africa at large. The '2014 outbreak' of the Ebola has been a major threat to not only Africa but the World at large. Ghana in this regard is no exception to the threats of Ebola Virus Disease (EVD) taking into cognizance that we are bounded by neighboring Ebola stricken Countries.

As the Ebola epidemic frenzies, two questions have surface: How did the noxious virus escape detection for three months? And why has a mammoth global interventions fail to contain it?

In Guinea, the case started in a small village (Meliandou) in the Forest region of southern Guinea. Bush meat has long been a common source of food for this village and they had it in bounty. But in the dying days of December the ordinary life in Meliandou came to an end when the Ebola virus gave a smooth landing in the village most likely in the body of a fruit bat-its natural non-human reservoir, according to a practical consensus among scientists. Ebola is one of the lethal viruses known to the world of Medical science, with no specific cure and mortality rates of up to 90 percent of affected people.

But the whodunit today is not how the epidemic began-it is why an unwavering attempt by an army of global connoisseur is being futile. Part of the answer is the chameleon-like character the virus displays in this part of the world. An even larger part lies in the global response itself. It was swift and comprehensive; exactly what you would anticipate. But there was a bewildering reaction that enervated everything the experts sought to achieve; and at the same time hoodwinked many of them into believing they had prospered in their aims. Finally they fathomed the truth. By then it was too late.

Jeffrey E. Stern reports that the outbreak started when a few tiny rod-shaped particles; each merely an attack plan, coded in ribonucleic acid and wrapped in a protein shell: found their way from a fruit bat into the body of a child not yet two years old. Perhaps, while the mother was preparing the day's hunt, some of the bat's blood was flung in the child's direction. Perhaps, while the mother's attention was elsewhere, the child touched the animal, then brought his hand to his mouth, the way babies do. Either way, a few strands of the Ebola virus attached themselves to cells in the child's immune system and used the cells' machinery to replicate. The boy developed a fever, then diarrhea and vomiting. His organs began to failing. He began to bleed internally and went into septic shock. In four days, he was dead

Until 2014, the deadliest Ebola outbreak on record had killed 280 people. As of this writing, 3,091 people have died from Ebola during the current West African outbreak, out of 6,574 confirmed cases, a report by World Health Organization (WHO). When Ebola strikes, it kills quickly, but it can take up to three weeks to incubate, and usually around 10 days.

Where Did It Originate? History of Ebola

The Ebola virus was first isolated and identified to 1976 in the Democratic Republic of Congo. This virus has been found to have an average mortality rate of 88 percent in humans, one of the highest recorded. Since its initial discovery, cases of Ebola fever have been identified and quarantined across central Africa.

The virus is spread by contact of bodily fluids and blood from others who are infected. Currently there are no documented cases of the virus spreading through the air. When this virus is contracted, individuals will start to show symptoms such as muscle pain, fever, headache or sore throat 2 days to 3 weeks later. This will be followed by rash, vomiting, diarrhea, decrease in kidney and liver function as well as internal and external bleeding. Prevention of these diseases focuses on decreasing the spread of the virus from animals to humans as there is not currently a treatment for this disease.

Ebola Virus Disease History

2014 Ebola Outbreak in West Africa

According to the most recent CDC outbreak information the countries of Nigeria, Guinea, Liberia and Sierra Leone are seeing one of the largest outbreaks of Ebola in world history. The Emergency Operations center is providing assistance and public health experts are working to expand resources to help control the outbreak. As of 20th August, more than 1400 people have died.

2012 Ebola Outbreak in Uganda (December)

In December 2012, 7 cases of Ebola were confirmed in the Luwero District of Uganda which caused 4 deaths. The Ministry of Health diagnosed and managed the outbreak with assistance from the Viral Special Pathogens Branch. The total numbers from this outbreak are expected to change.

2012 Ebola Outbreak in the Democratic Republic of Congo (November)

The DRC Ministry of Health declared an outbreak of Ebola in the Province Orientale on November 26, 2012. This outbreak included 77 cases confirmed by the CDC lab in Uganda which included 36 confirmed cases, 17 probable cases, 36 deaths and 24 suspected cases. The Public Health Agency of Canada provided additional diagnostic support for this outbreak.

2012 Ebola Outbreak in Uganda (July)

In July 2012, an outbreak of Ebola Hemorrhagic Fever in Kibaale Uganda was confirmed by the Uganda Ministry of Health. This included 24 probable human cases which are being researched at the Uganda Virus research Institute as well as the U.S. Centers for Disease Control and Prevention via blood sample. This outbreak has 11 confirmed patients with 4 deaths.

2011 Ebola Case in Uganda (May)

In May 2011 an outbreak of Ebola hemorrhagic fever was confirmed in the Luwero district of Uganda by the Ugandan Ministry of Health. Tests for the virus on blood samples confirmed the outbreak at the Uganda Viral Research Institute. To date, no additional cases have been reported.

2008 Ebola-Reston Virus Was Detected in Pigs in the Philippines

In October 2008 samples of tissue from pigs from the Philippines was tested by the Foreign Animal Disease Diagnostic Laboratory. These samples were taken from Manila where swine pathogens of the Ebola virus were identified using molecular analysis. This was the first time the Reston version of the virus was identified in pigs. An ongoing search is commencing to ensure that this virus was not spread to humans.

2007 Ebola Outbreak in the Democratic Republic of Congo

In August 2007 the Kasai Occidental Province was struck with a disease of unknown origins. Samples from the victims were sent to the CDC Special Pathogens Branch as well as the Centre International de Recherches Medicales de Franceville. Real time testing confirmed these cased to be from the Ebola virus, though the presence of other pathogens implies that additional diseases may have been present. This outbreak had a confirmed 249 cases resulting in 183 deaths.

2004 Ebola Outbreak in South Sudan

The World Health Organization confirmed 20 cases of Ebola hemorrhagic fever in Yambio County of south Sudan in 2004. This outbreak included 5 deaths which were studied by the Kenya Medical Research Institute and the Centers for Disease control. It was also confirmed that the strain which caused the outbreak was one previously known to cause human disease.

2003 Ebola Cases in the Democratic Republic of Congo

In 2003 several cases of Ebola hemorrhagic fever syndrome were confirmed by the World Health Organization Communicable Disease Surveillance and Response team in the Republic of the Congo.

2002 Ebola Outbreak in Gabon and Republic of the Congo

In May 2002, an outbreak of Ebola hemorrhagic fever was confirmed in the Ogooue Ivindo province by the Gabonese Ministry of Health and the World Health Organization. A response team was sent to this area and neighboring villages in the Republic of the Congo.

2001 Ebola Outbreak in Uganda

An outbreak of Ebola hemorrhagic fever which occurred over 42 days occurred in Uganda. It was officially declared over on February 27, 2001 after a period of time considered twice the maximum incubation period when no new cases were reported. Between October 2000-February 2001 the World Health Organization partnered with the CDC to help control the outbreak.

How Do You Get It?

To get Ebola, you need to have direct contact with the bodily fluids — such as vomit, urine, or blood — of someone who is already sick and symptomatic to get the disease.

But what, exactly, does that mean? Here is a more concrete guide on how the virus can move from one person to another.

How you can get Ebola

1) You can get the virus if you have "direct contact" with a range of bodily fluids from a sick person, including blood, saliva, breast milk, stool, sweat, semen, tears, vomit, and urine. "Direct contact" means these fluids need to get into your broken skin (such as a wound) or touch your mucous membranes (mouth, nose, eyes, vagina).

2) So you can get Ebola by kissing or sharing food with someone who is infectious.

3) Mothers with Ebola can give the disease to their babies. Ebola spreads through breastfeeding — even after recovery from the disease. As one study put it, "It seems prudent to advise breastfeeding mothers who survive (Ebola) to avoid breastfeeding for at least some weeks after recovery and to provide them with alternative means of feeding their infants."

4) You can get Ebola through sex with an Ebola patient. The virus has been able to live in semen up to 82 days after a patient became symptomatic, which means sexual transmission — even with someone who has survived the disease for months — is possible.

5) You can get the virus by eating wild animals infected with Ebola or coming into contact with their bodily fluids. The fruit bat is believed to be the animal reservoir for Ebola, and when its prepared for a meal or eaten raw, people get sick.

   So you can get the virus through exposure to bat secretions. However, if you cook a bat infected with Ebola and then eat it, you won't get sick because the virus dies during cooking.

6) You can get Ebola through contact with an infected surface. Though Ebola is easily killed with disinfectants like bleach, if it isn't caught, it can live outside the body on, say, a doorknob or counter top, for several hours. In body fluids, like blood, the virus can survive for several days. So you'd need to touch an infected surface, and then put your hands in your mouth and eyes.

   This is why the funerals of Ebola victims are problematic. Someone who has died from the virus will have a very high viral load. Since the virus can live in bodily fluids on their body, if you participate in the ritual washing of an Ebola victim and then touch your hands to your face, you could get the virus.

7) You could also get the virus by working in a Biosafety-level-4 lab that studies Ebola, touching lab specimens, and then putting your contaminated hands in your mouth, eyes or a cut.

8) You can get Ebola by being pricked with a needle or syringe that has been contaminated with the virus. This has been a source of transmission for health workers, but unless you're sharing needles with Ebola victims, this isn't likely.

What are the Signs and Symptoms?

The first case of Ebola diagnosed in the U.S. -- and news that health officials are monitoring as many as 100 people who may have come in direct or indirect contact with the patient in Dallas -- has further intensified fear of this deadly disease.

Public health officials have been clear about how it spreads: only through physical contact with the bodily fluids of an infected person who is showing symptoms of Ebola. It cannot be picked up through sneezing or coughing, like a cold or the flu.

What are the symptoms of Ebola, and how can doctors identify a patient who might have it before more people are put at risk of exposure?

The Centers for Disease Control and Prevention says these are the symptoms to watch out for:

- Fever (greater than 38.6°C or 101.5°F)
- Severe headache
- Muscle pain
- Weakness
- Diarrhea
- Vomiting
- Abdominal (stomach) pain
- Unexplained hemorrhage (bleeding or bruising)

The CDC says symptoms could start appearing anywhere from 2 to 21 days after exposure to the virus; the average incubation period is 8 to 10 days.

In the early stages of illness, symptoms like fever, headache and muscle pain are fairly common and may seem like a case of the flu.

However, within a few days, someone with Ebola will get much sicker. As the virus begins to take hold of the body, gastrointestinal illness, such as abdominal pain, vomiting and diarrhea will occur. A patient may have trouble breathing and swallowing, experience chest pain, and develop a rash, excessive bruising and bloody blisters of the skin.

A person in the advanced stages of an acute Ebola infection will begin to have internal bleeding -- what's known as viral hemorrhagic fever. Ebola can cause hemorrhaging of multiple organs, as well as external bleeding from various orifices of the body including the ears and eyes. While excessive bleeding is the most horrific of Ebola's symptoms, not every patient develops it.

Ebola has a mortality rate between 50 and 90 percent. People die from complications such as shock due to leaking of blood vessels. Other factors may be multiple organ failure, low blood pressure, jaundice, delirium, seizures and coma.

Health officials say it is not yet understood why some patients manage to recover, while so many others die. However, effective supportive care can make a big difference in the survival rate. These measures may include giving a patient intravenous fluids and electrolytes to counter dehydration caused by excessive vomiting and diarrhea; maintaining the patient's blood pressure; giving transfusions to replace blood lost due to hemorrhaging; as well as treating any subsequent infections that result from the virus.

"We depend of the body's defense to control the virus," explained Dr. Bruce Ribner, who specializes in infectious diseases at Emory University School of Medicine in Atlanta and led the team that treated two American aid workers who contracted the virus in Liberia over the summer. "We just have to keep the patient alive long enough, in order to survive the infection."

Know your enemy: It's hard to catch Ebola

Initial symptoms of Ebola are fever, sore throat, muscle and body aches, headaches, fatigue, vomiting and diarrhea. Sounds a lot like that flu bug you seem to catch at least once a year, right? But unlike the flu, Ebola does not spread through the air, meaning it's much harder to catch.

Ebola transmission requires contact between bodily fluids like vomit, blood, saliva, urine or sweat with your eyes, nose, mouth or broken skin. When the immune system begins breaking down, the symptoms begin to show. This process takes anywhere from two to 21 days (though it's typically between four to 10 days). (You can read more on how Ebola gets transmitted here.)

A key factor medical staff look for when someone wary of an Ebola infection goes to the hospital is the patient's travel history, like whether a person has recently spent time in one of the West African countries where the virus is widespread or with someone who has.

Influenza, on the other hand, is easily airborne on droplets projected from coughs and sneezes that fly through schools, offices and households, but can be prevented with the annual flu vaccine. The CDC advises people to cover their coughs and sneezes, wash their hands frequently, and recommends that caregivers and infants six months and older get the vaccine.

Ebola symptoms, if left untreated, usually intensify after eight to 12 days, whereas influenza symptoms tend to fade. But in rare cases, the flu can lead to severe symptoms.

"We have a vaccine and an antiviral medication for influenza, and it still causes deaths," said Dr. Mary Anne Jackson, the director of infectious diseases at Children's Mercy Hospital in Kansas City, Mo. "We have Americans afraid of Ebola, but fewer than 50 percent of Americans take advantage of the flu vaccine, and it's something that's going to be here. It's coming."

Who Do You Report to Once You Think You Have It?

When a Dallas County sheriff's deputy who had entered the apartment of the first patient to die from Ebola in the U.S. Started feeling ill himself, he didn't rush to the nearest hospital. He chose an urgent-care clinic.

So did a man who recently traveled to West Africa and was complaining of flu-like symptoms, prompting the suburban Boston urgent-care practice where he went to briefly shut down last week.

The deadly virus' arrival in the U.S. has put the spotlight on weak spots in American hospitals, but those facilities are not the only ones who have suddenly found themselves on the front lines against Ebola.

Urgent-care clinics for many people have become de facto emergency rooms. They are not, however, equipped like hospitals to treat serious illnesses, such as Ebola, nor do they have isolation units.

Clinics are urging potential patients to get checked for the highly contagious virus at a hospital.

Given the problems at the Texas hospital, where Thomas Eric Duncan died and two nurses have been diagnosed with the virus, an Ebola case could have posed even greater problems at a clinic or smaller hospital, experts say.

"That would be an even less controlled situation," said Dr. David Weber, an epidemiologist at the University of North Carolina's hospital. "The likelihood for that is so remote that they may never have thought about that."

Still, clinics are preparing staff in case someone with Ebola does walk in. They are distributing protective gear and quickly trying to get up to speed on the best protocols to teach their health providers.

Dr. William Gluckman of the Urgent Care Association of America, which represents more than 2,600 clinics, said the facilities want anyone who suspects they may have contracted Ebola to go to a hospital emergency department.

The Urgent Care Association of America sent emails to its roughly 6,400 members asking them to spread that message.

One of the fastest growing segments of the U.S. Health care industry with more than 9,000 clinics, urgent care is designed to treat as many patients as quickly as possible for minor illnesses, like the flu or a sliced finger.

But people are increasingly using them for any emergency to avoid the costs, long waits and crowds at hospitals.

"I think patients have a difficult time deciding where they need to go for care, so sometimes we'll see someone come in suffering from an acute heart attack or stroke, but urgent care shouldn't be the place to go for that," said Gluckman, who owns FastER urgent care clinic in Morris Plains, New Jersey.

MedExpress - which has 138 clinics in 11 states - said its employees have been told to encourage patients with flu-like symptoms who have been in West Africa or in contact with someone infected with Ebola to go to a hospital.

The Centers for Disease Control and Prevention says Ebola isn't contagious until symptoms appear. Ebola isn't spread through the air like the flu; people catch it by direct contact with a sick person's bodily fluids, such as blood or vomit.

The urgent care association recommends front desk staff ask for specifics on symptoms from patients and recent travel history.

If that the person has a fever, headache or other flu-like symptoms and has been in an Ebola hot spot, clinics have been told to isolate them in a single room, Gluckman said. The clinic should call public health officials and contact a hospital to transport them there as quickly as possible, per CDC guidelines.

Patients at the urgent care clinic in Frisco, a suburb north of Dallas, were held briefly after Dallas County sheriff's deputy Sgt. Michael Monning went there with flu-like symptoms. Monning had entered Duncan's apartment but had no direct contact with him.

Monning was transported to a hospital where it was determined that he did not have the virus.

Patients at the practice in Braintree, about 12 miles south of Boston, were also held briefly on Oct. 12 while the man who had been to West Africa was taken to a hospital, where it was determined he did not have Ebola. The car that he drove to the office was decontaminated by crews in hazmat suits.

CDC Director Tom Frieden said the agency is bolstering training nationwide on how to respond to an Ebola case.

U.S. health care has become more complex with retail clinics, urgent care centers, work-site clinics and even online clinics, so ensuring that everyone strictly follows protocol is going to continue to be a challenge.

But that's not necessarily a bad thing, said Dr. Tom Zweng of Novant Health, a four-state system based in Winston-Salem, North Carolina.

"This is not an exercise in futility," he said of the measures being taken to protect against Ebola. "This is preparing staff in safe practices. It may be Ebola today, but tomorrow there may be another communicable disease that we don't even know about. This is about taking health care in this country to the next level."

What are the Treatment Procedure?

There's no cure for Ebola, though researchers are working on it. Treatment includes an experimental serum that destroys infected cells.

Doctors manage the symptoms of Ebola with:

- Fluids and electrolytes
- Oxygen
- Blood pressure medication
- Blood transfusions
- Treatment for other infections

WHO aims for Ebola serum in weeks and vaccine tests in Africa by January. Details given of two vaccines being fast-tracked for trial on 20,000 health workers and antibody serum planned for Liberia.

A volunteer receives the Ebola vaccination at the vaccine center in Bamako, Mali. Photograph: Alex Duval Smith/dpa/Corbis.

The World Health Organization has announced it hopes to begin testing two experimental Ebola vaccines in West Africa by January and may have a blood serum treatment available for use in Liberia within two weeks.

The UN's health agency said it aimed to begin testing the two vaccines in the new year on more than 20,000 frontline health care workers and others in West Africa – a bigger rollout than previously envisioned.

Separately, a senior Red Cross official said he was confident the epidemic could be contained within four to six months.

Elhadj As Sy, the secretary general of the International Federation of Red Cross and Red Crescent Societies, told reporters in Beijing on Wednesday that the outbreak could be contained if there was "good isolation, good treatment of the cases which are confirmed, good dignified and safe burials of deceased people."

Dr Marie Paule Kieny, an assistant director general at the WHO, said the first tens of thousands of Ebola vaccines could be distributed in the first months of the new year. Kieny acknowledged there were many "ifs" remaining and "still a possibility that it [a vaccine] will fail". But she sketched out a much broader experiment than was imagined only six months ago.

"These are quite large trials," she said.

Kieny said in remarks reported by the BBC that a serum was also being developed for use in Liberia based on antibodies extracted from the blood of Ebola survivors. "There are partnerships which are starting to be put in place to have capacity in the three countries to safely extract plasma and make preparation that can be used for the treatment of infective patients.

"The partnership which is moving the quickest will be in Liberia where we hope that in the coming weeks there will be facilities set up to collect the blood, treat the blood and be able to process it for use."

A WHO spokeswoman, Fadela Chaib, said the agency expected 20,000 vaccinations in January and similar numbers in the months afterwards using the trial products.

An effective vaccine would still not in itself be enough to stop the outbreak but could protect the medical workers who are central to the effort. More than 200 of them have died of Ebola.

The real-world testing in West Africa will go forward only if the vaccines prove safe and trigger an adequate immune-system response in volunteers during clinical trials that are either under way or planned in Europe, Africa and the US. The preliminary safety data is expected to become available by December.

One of the vaccines that Kieny mentioned, Okairos AG, is being developed by the US National Institutes of Health and GlaxoSmithKline from a modified chimpanzee-cold virus and an Ebola protein. It is being made in Rome, according to GSK, with clinical trials under way in Britain and Mali.

"We have other vaccine facilities around the world and we are seeing what we can do to ramp up production to commercial scale," said Mary Anne Rhyne, GSK's US director of external communications.

The second frontrunner, developed by the Public Health Agency of Canada and known as VSV-EBOV, has been sent to the US Walter Reed Army Institute of Research in Maryland for testing on healthy volunteers. It would also be tested shortly among volunteers in Switzerland, Germany, Gabon and Kenya, Kieny said.

Separately, the Canadian drugmaker Tekmira Pharmaceuticals announced on Tuesday it had begun limited manufacturing of a therapeutic product targeting the Ebola-Guinea virus.

Tekmira said on Tuesday that the new product, part of its TKM-Ebola programme, would be available by early December. But it did not specify how many doses it was making, or whether it was a drug or vaccine. Its TKM-Ebola program is aimed at developing a treatment to stop the virus replicating in an infected person.

The European Medicines Agency said on Monday it was ready to offer Ebola treatments and vaccines the benefits of "orphan" drug status – including extended market exclusivity – in a bid to encourage their development.

Mapp Biopharmaceutical – which gave its experimental Ebola treatment ZMapp to US medical workers Dr Kent Brantly and Nancy Writebol, who recovered after contracting Ebola in Liberia, and to at least one Spanish priest, who died – said it had begun manufacturing the drug using conventional methods that would produce greater quantities for more human testing.

The outbreak in west Africa has killed more than 4,500 people, mostly in Liberia, Guinea and Sierra Leone, since it began 10 months ago. Experts have said the world could see 10,000 new cases a week in two months if authorities did not take stronger steps.

Are You Going to Die If You Contract the Virus?

There's no cure for Ebola. So why have some patients walked away healthy while others in the West died?

Dr. Kent Brantly, Nancy Writebol and Dr. Rick Sacra all contracted the disease while working in Liberia -- and all survived.

Spanish nurse's aide Teresa Romero Ramos got the virus while tending to stricken patients. She too lived.

But like the patients above, Thomas Eric Duncan and Spanish priest Miguel Pajares also received treatment in the West. Yet they died.

Blair: Ebola crisis is extremely serious

While there might not be a single, conclusive answer, a series of factors may contribute to survival. Relatives afraid to take in Ebola orphans.

Early, High-Quality Treatment

This may be the most critical factor in beating Ebola.

The survivors in the United States all have one thing in common -- they were rushed to two of the country's four hospitals that have been preparing for years to treat a highly infectious disease such as Ebola.

Brantly and Writebol were successfully treated at Emory University Hospital in Atlanta; Sacra was released from the Nebraska Medical Center in Omaha.

Duncan didn't go to one of those four hospitals. He went to Texas Health Presbyterian Hospital in Dallas with a fever and told them he'd recently returned from Liberia. Yet the hospital initially sent him home with antibiotics.

Then, after he returned to the hospital much more ill, two nurses became sick with the virus. They have since been moved to more specialized facilities such as Emory and the National Institutes of Health in Maryland.

But that doesn't mean patients are doomed just because they go to a different hospital.

"Keep in mind that this is still a very deadly disease," said Dr. Sanjay Gupta, CNN's chief medical correspondent. "In West Africa, the mortality rates are above 60%. I think it is better in the United States. But they're not going to be zero, I think no matter where somebody is."

Quick Rehydration

After finding a hospital capable of treating Ebola, those who survive are usually rehydrated quickly.

"The most important care of patients with Ebola is to manage their fluids and electrolytes, to make sure that they don't get dehydrated," said Dr. Tom Frieden, director of the Centers for Disease Control and Prevention. "And that requires some meticulous attention to detail and aggressive rehydration in many cases."

And if an infected patient getting proper care normally has a strong immune system, the chance of surviving goes up.

But what may seem basic in the United States can be difficult to come by in West Africa, where Ebola has already killed more than 4,500 people -- largely because access to health care is limited.

Yet Nigeria has successfully eradicated Ebola from the country, the World Health Organization said Monday.

Unlike in Guinea, Liberia and Sierra Leone -- the combined epicenter of the outbreak -- all identified contacts in Nigeria were physically monitored every day for 21 days, WHO said.

Plasma Transfusions

Three Ebola patients -- Sacra, NBC cameraman Ashoka Mukpo and Texas nurse Nina Pham -- all received plasma donations from Brantly. And all three have survived.

The theory is that Brantly's plasma contains the antibodies necessary to fight the virus.

"It's very fortunate that the three patients I've been able to donate to, they and I share the same blood type," Brantly told CNN's Anderson Cooper.

"I'll keep doing it as much as it's needed, as much as I can."

There was some controversy about why Brantly didn't give plasma to Duncan. But the problem came down to blood type, Texas Health Presbyterian Hospital said.

WHO to review Ebola response amid criticism of its efforts.

Experimental Drugs

Medication that hasn't gone through clinical trials can be risky. But with a mortality rate of 50% in the current Ebola outbreak, a WHO panel said it is ethical to offer drugs to fight the virus - even if their effectiveness or adverse effects are unknown.

The experimental drugs at the center of this Ebola outbreak are ZMapp, Favipiravir, Brincidofovir and TKM-Ebola.

Brantly and Writebol both took ZMapp, and both survived. But Pajares also took ZMapp, and he died.

The director of Emory's Infectious Disease Unit cautioned against viewing ZMapp as a surefire cure.

"They are the very first individuals to have ever received this agent," Dr. Bruce Ribner said. "There is no prior experience with it, and frankly, we do not know whether it helped them, whether it made no difference, or even, theoretically, if it delayed their recovery."

Spanish nurse's aide Teresa Romero Ramos took the anti-viral drug Favipiravir and also received antibodies from a survivor in West Africa. She is now free of the virus.

In addition to getting a blood transfusion, Sacra received an experimental drug called TKM-Ebola, which the Food and Drug Administration recently approved for wider use.

Duncan took a different untested drug, Brincidofovir. But he didn't receive it until six days after being admitted to the Texas hospital. Had he taken it earlier, the outcome might have been different.

How Long Does the Sickness Last?

The Ebola virus disease originally appeared on the world stage in 1976 when not one, but two simultaneous outbreaks hit two different areas in Africa. Over the next three and a half decades around 2000 people were killed by this deadly virus. Now, if you have been watching the news lately you know that a new Ebola outbreak is currently ravaging West Africa. Even with a lower mortality rate of only about 60% compared to as high as 90% in previous outbreaks, over 2500 people have already lost their lives, making this the deadliest Ebola virus outbreak in world history. Three American hospitals, located in New York City, have had to isolate and test potential Ebola cases already with the most recent case at Mount Sinai Hospital in Manhattan. All patients presented with early Ebola-like symptoms and several had recently traveled in West Africa. Fortunately, according to the New York Times, none of these individuals tested positive for the virus.

However, if people do get infected with the Ebola virus, what are the chances of recovering from this disease and how long does this process last?

What Are the Chances of Recovering from Ebola?

The World Health Organization (WHO) states that the Ebola virus is "a severe, often fatal illness, with a case fatality rate of up to 90%." However, the death rate can be as low as 50% if prompt diagnosis is made the proper supportive care/ treatment is given.

The early symptoms include, but are not limited to; sudden onset of fever, generalized weakness, muscle pains, chills, headaches and sore throat. As the disease progresses the symptoms grow worse, including nausea, vomiting, diarrhea, bloody stool, bloodshot eyes, rash, chest pain and coughing, stomach pain, severe and rapid weight loss, bruising, bleeding from various orifices (usually the eyes), internal bleeding, impaired kidney function and impaired liver function.

The Ebola virus is transmitted by direct contact with infected blood, bodily fluids and tissue of infected people or animals (alive or dead) and with an incubation period of as little as two days (or as many as 21), people remain infections as long as their blood and fluids contain the virus.

With no known cure (several are in testing) for the disease, the only treatments available are labeled as "supportive intensive care" and are administered to treat the symptoms and provide some small level of comfort. During outbreaks, the people who are most at risk are health care workers, family members and any others who come into close and/or frequent contact with infected individuals, alive or deceased.

How Long Does It Take to Recover from Ebola?

While the chances of surviving the Ebola virus if one becomes infected are slim, there are those are able to weather the storm and survive their near brush with death. The question then is: if I survive, how long will it take to recover?

To answer that we will turn to Dr. Tim Lahey, M.D. (an infectious disease specialist and professor of medicine as well as microbiology and immunology with Dartmouth's Geisel School of Medicine. When asked how long it would take someone to clinically recover from the Ebola virus, Dr. Lahey stated that you could expect a few week recovery time. It generally takes one to two weeks for symptoms of the disease to appear, on average, and from that point death generally occurs within a couple of weeks. If you are lucky enough to survive, after this few week period you could be considered as recovered.

Case 1 of Recovery from Ebola

Twenty-seven year old Fanta battled this terrible disease for weeks, horrified that she had become infected with a disease which could not be cured. Hailing from Guinea,

Fanta had contracted the most severe strain of Ebola, known as Zaire Ebola, which in previous outbreaks held a mortality rate of 90 percent.

Due to her "extraordinary capacity for resistance", Fanta achieved what most stricken with the Ebola virus cannot... she lived! Now known as the miracle woman who survived Ebola, onlookers crowd around Fanta when she spoke of her ordeal and bombarded medical staff with questions about how she managed it.

The doctors from Doctors Without Borders state that chances of survival are greatly increased if the patient is kept hydrated and all symptoms and secondary infections treated. As for Fanta, she simply says that "It is as if I have just been reborn".

Case 2 of Recovery from Ebola

Twenty-nine year old Abdullah first came to the doctors at a hospital close to his home in Conakry in late March presenting with a high fever, headaches and weakness. Due to the Ebola virus outbreak, the doctor quickly called in infections disease experts and transferred Abdullah to an isolation facility in Donka. Once there, Abdullah was tested and found to be positive for Ebola. He was devastated.

With 10 days spent in the isolation facility, Abdullah, father of twins, was confident he would never again see his wife or children. After battling the disease for five days, his condition began to improve. The fever went down, the diarrhea and vomiting went away, the bleeding stopped. The doctors took a new blood sample and miraculously it came back negative for Ebola.

Much like our miracle woman, Fanta, Abdullah says "I felt as if I was reborn". He was able to return to his wife and to hug his twins again. Abdullah credits his recovery to the wonderful doctors who took care of him during his illness and recommends anyone infected with Ebola go to the facility where he was treated.

What Lies Ahead for Those Who Survived Ebola?

For those lucky few who survive the battle with Ebola the question remains, what comes next? While most survivors are able to go back to their day to day lives there are still a few concerns. We are not 100 percent sure how long they may still be able to pass the virus along. Estimations range from a few weeks to a few months. During this time, extra precautions must be taken, such as wearing a condom during intercourse.

They are also more prone to develop chronic inflammatory conditions affecting both the joints and eyes. In the joints, survivors are at risk for arthralgia which feels similar to arthritis and in the eyes they often come down with uveitis which at best causes sensitivity and excessive tearing...at worst, blindness.

What are the Side Effects of the Medicine?

While most of the recent coverage of the ongoing Ebola outbreak has focused on rising death tolls and a few infected U.S. Citizens, other segments of the population have passed mostly unnoticed from the harsh glare of the media spotlight: Survivors, and those who are seemingly immune to Ebola.

People who survive Ebola can lead normal lives post-recovery, though occasionally they can suffer inflammatory conditions of the joints afterwards, according to CBS. Recovery times can vary, and so can the amount of time it takes for the virus to clear out of the system. The World Health Organization found that the virus can reside in semen for up to seven weeks after recovery. Survivors are generally assumed to be immune to the particular strain they are infected by, and are able to help tend to others infected with the same strain. What isn't clear is whether or not a person is immune to other strains of Ebola, or if their immunity will last.

As with most viral infections, patients who recover from Ebola end up with Ebola-fighting antibodies in their blood, making their blood a valuable (if controversial) treatment option for others who catch the infection. Kent Brantly, one of the most recognizable Ebola survivors, has donated more than a gallon of his blood to other patients. The plasma of his blood, which contains the antibodies, is separated out from the red blood cells, creating what's known as a convalescent serum, which can then be given to a patient as a transfusion. The hope is that the antibodies in the serum will boost the patient's immune response, attacking the virus, and allowing the body to recover.

But this treatment method, like all Ebola treatment methods, is far from ideal. To start with, scientists aren't even sure if it works. In addition, the serum can only be donated to people with a compatible blood type to the donor, and it's unclear how long the immunity would last. Adding to the confusion, there are several different strains of

Ebola, and there's no guarantee that once someone has recovered from one strain of Ebola they are immune to others.

When Nancy Writebol, one of the survivors of Ebola who was whisked back to Atlanta soon after contracting the virus, was asked by Science Magazine if she would consider going back, she said:

"I've done some reading on that and talked to doctors at Emory about that. My doctors at Emory are not sure how long immunity would last. It's not been studied. I've read that even if a survivor was willing and able to help with the care for Ebola patients, because there are so many strains of Ebola, it would still be very wise and necessary to operate in PPEs and not just assume you're immune."

People who survived the disease are of particular interest to researchers, such as those working on the ZMapp drug, who hope that they can synthesize antibodies in the hopes of creating a cure.

But even less understood than the survivors are the people who were infected with Ebola but never developed any symptoms. After outbreaks in Uganda in the late 1990's, scientists tested the blood of several people who were in close contact with Ebola patients, and found a number of them had markers in their blood indicating they carried the disease, but they were totally asymptomatic—they managed to completely avoid the horrifying symptoms of the disease.

In a letter in the Lancet this week, researchers look into the existence of these asymptomatic patients, and hope that identifying people who are naturally immune could help contain the outbreak as scientists work on developing a treatment. A 2010 study published by the French research organization IRD found that as much as 15.3 percent of Gabon's population could be immune to Ebola.

"Ultimately, knowing whether a large segment of the population in the afflicted regions are immune to Ebola could save lives," Steve Bellan, an author of the Lancet letter, said in a press release. "If we can reliably identify who they are, they could become people who help with disease-control tasks, and that would prevent exposing others who aren't immune. We might not have to wait until we have a vaccine to use immune individuals to reduce the spread of disease."

Being able to reliably identify naturally immune patients is still a ways off, but Bellan and his fellow researchers hope that by studying the current outbreak and looking for asymptomatic individuals, they might be able to save lives in the future.

How Do You Protect Yourself from Getting It?

1) You can't get Ebola from someone who is not already sick. The virus only turns up in people's bodily fluids after a person starts to feel ill, and only then can they spread it to another person.

2) You can't get Ebola from mosquitoes. The CDC says, "Only mammals (for example, humans, bats, monkeys and apes) have shown the ability to spread and become infected with Ebola virus."

3) You usually can't get Ebola through coughing or sneezing. The virus isn't airborne, thankfully, and experts expect that it will never become airborne. But, the Centers for Disease Control and Prevention said, "If a symptomatic patient with Ebola coughs or sneezes on someone, and saliva or mucus come into contact with that person's eyes, nose or mouth, these fluids may transmit the disease." This happens rarely and usually only affects health workers or those caring for the sick.

The bottom line: Ebola is difficult to catch

Ebola isn't very easy to transmit. The scenarios under which it spreads are very specific. And Ebola doesn't spread quickly, either. A mathematical epidemiologist who studies Ebola wrote in the Washington Post, "The good news is that Ebola has a lower reproductive rate than measles in the pre-vaccination days or the Spanish flu." He found that each Ebola case produces between 1.3 and 1.8 secondary cases. That means an Ebola victim usually only infects about one other person. Compare that with measles, which creates 17 secondary cases.

If you do the math, that means a single case in the US could lead to one or two others — which is exactly what has happened in the US so far with the Dallas situation. Because we have robust public health measures here, it probably won't go further than that. Compare that to West Africa, which is now dealing with upwards of 8,000 cases in a completely broken health system. That's where experts say the worry about Ebola should be placed.

How do you protect yourself from getting it?

If you have recently travelled to an area that has been affected by Ebola or have come into contact with someone who may at risk, there are several ways of limiting your chance of catching the virus

Ebola is spread by contact with the fluids of someone who is infected with Ebola, including saliva, sweat, blood and vomit. No vaccine or cure is available.

If you have recently travelled to an area that has been affected, such as Liberia, Guinea or Sierra Leone, or have come into contact with someone who may at risk, there are several ways of limiting your chance of catching Ebola.

Despite the seriousness of the disease, which causes bleeding from the mouth, ears and eyes, preventing it spreading is relatively simple.

According to the Centre for Disease Control and Prevention, it is important to wash your hands thoroughly with warm water and soap or, if that is not available, a hand sanitiser can be used.

Avoid any contact with someone you believe is infected, especially with their bodily fluids, advises the World Health Organisation (WHO).

If you need to go near someone with the virus, use protective gear such as face masks and gloves.

Health workers in West Africa have taken full precautions, wearing protective suits that cover their entire bodies, as well as hosing down areas infected patients have used.

WHO states any areas an infected person could have had contact with, such as bed linens, should be disinfected.

If you believe someone you know has been infected, or if you think you might have contracted Ebola, the best thing to do is isolate yourself from any other people around you and call medical help immediately.

A sudden temperature, muscle aches, vomiting or a rash might indicates you have the disease.

Is There a Possibility for It to Be Used in a Bioterrorism?

Ebola's exponential spread has rekindled fears that terrorists may seek to turn the virus into a powerful weapon of mass destruction. Such talk has occurred on Capitol Hill and in national security circles. But the financial and logistical challenges of transforming Ebola into a tool of bioterror makes the concern seem overblown—at least as far as widespread devastation is concerned.

National security and infectious disease experts agree the obstacles to a large-scale assault with Ebola are formidable. For starters, a bioterrorist would have to obtain the virus and be able to grow a massive supply in large vats, an extremely costly endeavor. While the virus is easily spread through personal contact with the bodily fluids of an infected person, it would be difficult to manipulate and control. Put simply, a large amount of Ebola in the hands of a rogue group would more likely end up killing the plotters than making it to the endgame of a bioterrorism mission. To be successful, "it would take a state-type [agent]" with more extensive resources, Anthony Fauci, the director of the National Institute of Allergy and Infectious Diseases, told a Congressional committee last week.

Already there is historical precedent for states trying—and failing—to tap the virus for bioterror. During the Cold War, the Soviet Union was "growing up large amounts of microbes for potential use in bioterrorism. That was known through intelligence," Fauci told Scientific American. The Soviets attempted to cultivate smallpox, anthrax, tularemia, botulism and hemorrhagic fevers including Ebola, he says. Yet exactly how the country would have deployed the microbes remains an area of speculation. The Soviets eventually dropped the project, but they were not the only ones interested in the microbe's potential.

The Japanese cult Aum Shinrikyo—infamous for setting off sarin gas in a Tokyo subway in 1995—also looked into Ebola as a potential biological weapon. In 1992, they sent a medical group of 40 people ostensibly to help provide aid during an Ebola outbreak in the Democratic Republic of the Congo. Their real purpose, however, was to collect some Ebola virus, as Amy Smithson, a senior fellow at the James Martin Center for Nonproliferation Studies, noted in her 2000 report Ataxia. The effort was a "flagrant failure," she says. "They did not get their hands on a culture."

Even if Aum Shinrikyo had managed to gather samples of the Ebola virus, it would have been extremely difficult to kill large numbers of people in countries with a strong health infrastructure such as Japan. Once the virus had been identified and patients isolated, the pathogen would have been unlikely to spread widely. Still, any terrorist attempting to stoke fears rather than accrue a high body count could have some modicum of success with Ebola. "When talking about bioterror, it's more about the terror than it is the bio," Fauci says.

Interviews with Fauci and other infection and security experts suggest that the virus could potentially be used for small-scale Ebola attacks in about three different ways—although each approach would run up against substantial logistical, financial and biological barriers. First, Ebola could be weaponized by taking large quantities of it and inserting them into a small "bomblet" that, once detonated, would spray the virus perhaps 30 feet—potentially infecting people as it landed on their faces, on cuts or on hands that they might then touch their eyes with. "That would be like a hundred people simultaneously touching an Ebola-infected person," says Fauci. Ebola would not need to be altered in any way to make such a plot work. The virus is already so capable of spreading from person to person via contact with bodily fluids that in its natural state it could do some serious damage. "Ebola is a very lethal pathogenic virus," says virologist Robert Garry of Tulane University. "It's basically weaponizing itself."

The second, and perhaps easiest, small-scale bioterrorism option would be to recruit individuals for Ebola suicide missions. Such a plan would hinge on injecting Ebola virus into a limited number of people, who would then need to leave west Africa (or wherever the outbreak may be) before becoming symptomatic. Then those individuals would have to get into a public space and projectile vomit or bleed onto others to infect them. Obviously the plot would need to overcome substantial technical challenges, including the extreme weakness that arises from Ebola. If it did succeed, this mode of transmission would not kill thousands of people, but it would set off significant fears.

The third bioterrorism method appears to be the most unlikely: genetically modifying the virus to enable it to spread more readily, perhaps through the air. As Scientific American reported on September 16, transforming the Ebola virus from a pathogen that primarily affects the circulatory system to one well suited for the respiratory system would be a major research undertaking. While theoretically the microbe could be manipulated to act in that way, it would be a demanding choice for nefarious actors looking to stockpile harmful materials.

With an Ebola outbreak that has already killed more than 2,800 in West Africa and laid siege to the health care systems of Guinea, Liberia and Sierra Leone, it is clear that already Ebola is terrorizing thousands. Nevertheless, the possibility of rogue organizations sowing this terror on a similar scale seems largely out of reach.

Conclusion

Thank you again for downloading this book!

I hope this book was able to help you to better understand Ebola virus - its origin, its strength, and how would we be able to get in contact with them. Most importantly, this book clearly state how do we protect ourselves from getting the virus.

The next step is to start implementing the tips you have learned from the book so you can get a worry-free healthy life.

Finally, if you enjoyed this book, please take the time to share your thoughts and post a review on Amazon. It'd be greatly appreciated!

Thank you and good luck!

Review Link

If you enjoyed this book, we would really appreciate it if you could leave us a positive REVIEW?

P.S. **You can <u>CLICK HERE</u> to go directly to the book page** and leave your review and/or purchase our other books above. Alternatively, you can copy and paste this address into your browser --- http://amzn.to/1wCj3OE

Preview of Gout Cure
Your Ultimate and Comprehensive Guide in Treating Gout Permanently

Gout is an inflammatory type of arthritis. It is characterized by severe pain, tenderness and swelling of the affected part. It often affects the big toe, that's about half of the cases of gout, however, it also affects the other parts of the body such as joints and some muscles.

Disease of the Kings

It is caused by the excess uric acid in the blood that gets accumulated in the joints of the body forming crystals. Uric acid comes from purine rich food such as meat, poultry and fatty fish. Gout could be traced in the olden times and often referred to as the "disease of the kings." Why? Because during those times there are many foods that only those who are in the higher level of society can afford. Chocolate is one example, some ale and meats are also consumed largely on banquets.

King Henry VIII of England is probably the most popular king to have suffered from gout. He was always depicted in pictures or paintings as someone holding a chunk of meat in one hand and a drink on the other. He was also obese which increases the risk of having gout.

Stages of Gout

There are said to be four stages of gout, which are Asymptomatic, Acute, Interval and Chronic Tophaceous. The first stage, asymptomatic is characterized by increased levels of uric acid in blood, however, there is no other symptoms, such as pain or swelling present in the patient. The Acute gout stage is characterized by intense pain which is brought about by the uric acid deposits. It can last for days, but will subside even without treatment. The interval stage is the period between attacks. In this stage, there are no symptoms experienced, like the asymptomatic stage, the uric acid level is still elevated and the chances of having a following attack are at a much higher risk. The chronic tophaceous gout is developed over a long period of time. In this stage tophi may have already developed into skin and in soft tissues.

Tophi is a mass of uric acid crystals. It forms in the skin and around the joints or on the tips of the fingers as nodes. It is considered to be a manifestation of gout in of the advanced stage. Although it usually forms around the joints, it may form just about anywhere in the body. It is also sometimes referred to as chalkstones because of its white, chalk-like appearance.

If you like this preview, then *click here for the full story of this eBook!*

Or go to: *http://www.amazon.com/dp/B00VB1428S/*

Check Out My Other Books

Ultimate Guide to Financial Freedom: Achieve Wealth, Attain Success, and Manage your Debt Like the Rich!

Dedication

To our three blessings that have made RicTamily complete and continue to grow together in His loving embrace.

Disclaimer

The information in this book is in no way intended as medical advice. This book is not meant to be used, nor should it be used, to diagnose or treat any medical condition. The author disclaims responsibility for any adverse health effects that come in combination with the use of methods and suggestions presented in the book. The publisher and author are not responsible for any health or allergy needs that may require medical supervision and are not liable for any damages or negative consequences from any treatment, action, application or preparation, to any person reading or following the information in this book.

www.ingramcontent.com/pod-product-compliance
Lightning Source LLC
Chambersburg PA
CBHW040926180526
45159CB00002BA/627